TOP FITNESS ADVICE

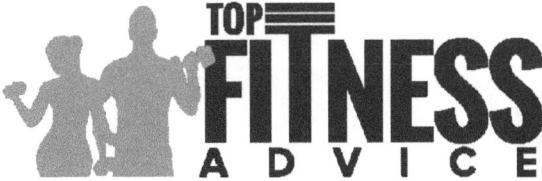

EAT TO LIVE DIET

How You Can Hack Healthy Eating
& Nutrition To Achieve Fast Weight
Loss That You Never Gain Back

Bruce Harlow

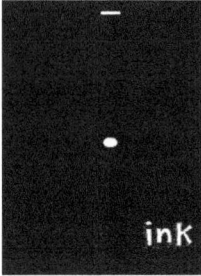

First published in 2017 by Venture Ink Publishing

Copyright © Top Fitness Advice 2019

For more information about the contents of this book or questions to the author, please contact Bruce Harlow at bruce@topfitnessadvice.com

Disclaimer

This book provides wellness management information in an informative and educational manner only, with information that is general in nature and that is not specific to you, the reader. The contents of this book are intended to assist you and other readers in your personal wellness efforts. Consult your physician regarding the applicability of any information provided in this book to you.

Nothing in this book should be construed as personal advice or diagnosis, and must not be used in this manner. The information provided about conditions is general in nature. This information does not cover all possible uses, actions, precautions, side-effects, or interactions of medicines, or medical procedures. The information in this book should not be considered as complete and does not cover all diseases, ailments, physical conditions, or their treatment.

You should consult with your physician before beginning any exercise, weight loss, or health care program. This book should not be used in place of a call or visit to a competent health-care professional. You should consult a health care professional before adopting any of the suggestions in this book or before drawing inferences from it.

Any decision regarding treatment and medication for your condition should be made with the advice and consultation of a qualified health care professional. If you have, or suspect you have, a health-care problem, then you should immediately contact a qualified health care professional for treatment.

No Warranties: The author and publisher don't guarantee or warrant the quality, accuracy, completeness, timeliness, appropriateness or suitability of the information in this book, or of any product or services referenced in this book.

The information in this book is provided on an "as is" basis and the author and publisher make no representations or warranties of any kind with respect to this information. This book may contain inaccuracies, typographical errors, or other errors.

Table of Contents

Would you prefer to listen to my book, rather than read it?

Download the audiobook version for free!

If you go to the special link below and sign up to Audible as a new customer, you can get the audiobook version of my book completely free.

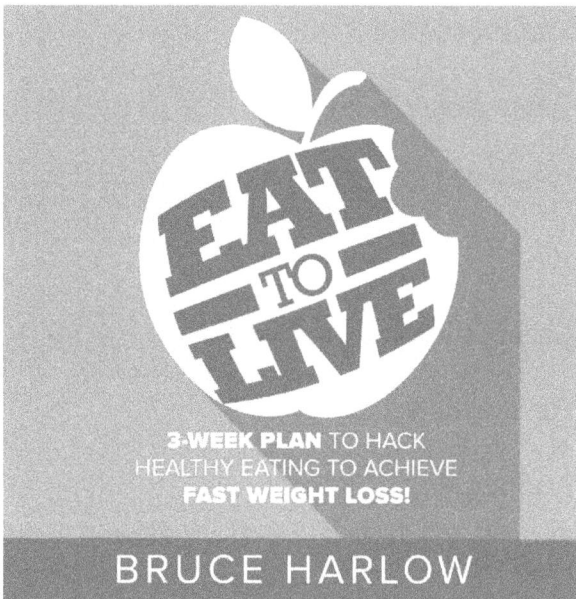

Go here to get your audiobook version for free:

TopFitnessAdvice.com/go/EatDiet

Who is this book for?

This book is meant to be for people who struggle with healthy eating and are looking for a route to change their ways throughout the duration of their life. This book is meant to be for people who aren't interested in going on a diet, rather they are interested in changing their whole lifestyle for the better.

This book is meant for people who are willing to work hard throughout their life and people who are tired of following the same diet's that never work out for them. The main goal of this book is to lose your weight as fast as possible, but also to keep it off forever as well and this is not an easy task by any means.

This book is meant for someone who has tried and tried to lose weight; maybe even successfully at times, but they haven't managed to keep it off. It takes dedication and a lifetime commitment and some people just aren't cut out for doing that much work in order to have a healthy body that they enjoy living in.

If you are willing to eat healthy for the rest of your life, keep track of what you eat for the rest of your life and live and feel better for the rest of your life then this book was written just for you, after reading this book you will be able to hack nutrition healthy eating to lose weight and get the body you desire.

What will this book teach you?

This book will teach you the things that you should eat in order to lose weight fast and never gain it back. Luckily, this book is not meant to just be a quick weight loss method. It is in fact made with the goal of maintaining a healthy lifestyle throughout your life.

It can be really difficult to lose weight fast if you don't know what you are doing. This book will teach you how to properly count calories as well as teach you about some of the other things that you may not have thought about on ingredient labels that can have an impact on your health.

This book will help to show you how to maintain a balanced lifestyle so that you can keep your weight off and yet enjoy the food that you eat. It will teach you the importance of size portions as well as rationing your calories so that you can make it through the day without becoming hungry.

This book will teach you methods to help make you feel better about yourself and get you on track for a healthy life. It is important to keep in mind that although this book should be exactly what you need to start having a healthy life, disease and problems affect even the best of us at times and it can be impossible to avoid.

Introduction

If you want to be able to lose weight successfully, you are going to really have to put your mind to it. The problem with most diets is that they put you on a plan that is impossible to follow.

Most diets don't allow you to eat the foods that you want to eat and most diets don't allow you to adapt you're eating styles and are much more of a temporary fix than that of what you should actually be looking for.

In order to lose the weight that you want to lose you are going to have to be ready to make sacrifices not just during the 21-day challenge that this diet puts you through, but for the rest of your life. Losing weight fast is difficult and it requires a lot of effort.

It is important to realize that each and every day you have the potential to lose or gain weight. The amount that you gain may be extremely minimal, but generally speaking you are either losing weight or gaining weight on a daily basis depending on the needs of your body on that particular day as well as how many calories you are consuming.

It is also important to realize that your metabolism does play a large part in how quickly you are able to burn calories and therefore lose weight. The more muscle mass that you have in your body, the more calories your body is going to burn just to be able to feed those muscles with the proper nutrition and calories that they need to thrive.

Another thing that certainly plays a role in your weight loss is the times of day that you eat. If you eat most of your calories in the morning then your body has the entire day to burn these calories off. Meanwhile if you are eating a lot of calories at night, your body won't be able to use the calories for much and will store the calories as fat accordingly so that the calories/ energy can be used at a later date.

There is a large debate over which types of ingredients offer the best weight loss and generally speaking it isn't all that important to you. Just make sure that your body is getting the proper nutrition that it needs each and every day and set your calorie goals and combine fitness as well as good eating habits so that you are able to reach your goals at a faster rate.

Did You Know You Are MOST Likely Burning Fat Too SLOW?

Discover The Most POWERFUL Method to Start Burning Fat Up to 400% Faster!

For this month only, you can get Bruce's best-selling & most popular book absolutely free – *The Most Powerful Method to Burn Fat Up to 400% Faster!*

Get Your FREE Copy Here:

TopFitnessAdvice.com/Download

Discover exactly what you need to do to **put your metabolism into hyperdrive** and have your **fat melt away effortlessly**. And learn the biological "hacks" that have been scientifically proven to **boost the rate that your body burns fat by up to 400%.** With this book, readers were able to reach their fitness goals significantly quicker, so it's highly recommended that you get this book, especially while it's free!

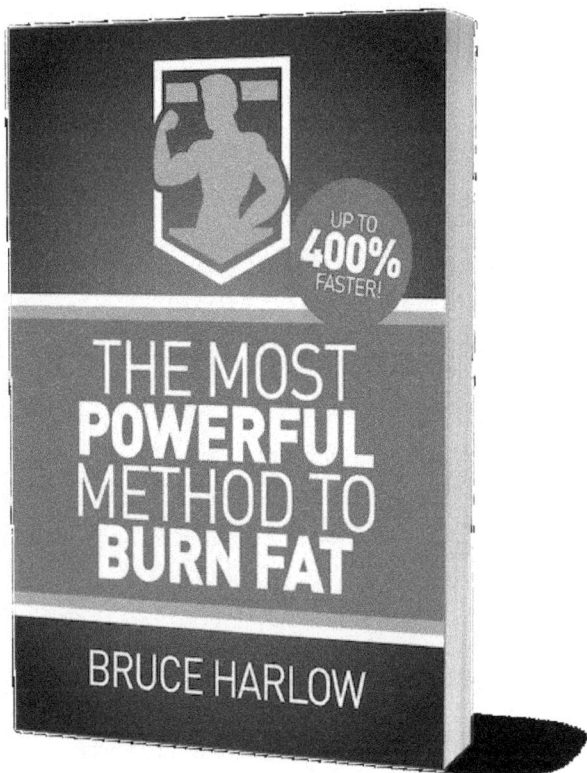

Get Your FREE Copy Here:

TopFitnessAdvice.com/Download

Chapter 1

Losing the Weight - Getting Started

The best way to lose weight and never gain it back is to lose it at a fast rate, and then continue to monitor your calorie intake and eat under the daily recommended amount of calories for your body type.

You should never go by the daily 2000 calorie recommendation on the back of the package, instead you should look up your body type and activity level in order to see the amount of calories that your unique body will consume on its own on a daily basis.

The amount of calories naturally burned by a person can vary a lot depending on their body type and physical activity. Make sure that you answer honestly as lying during this process will only damage yourself and your weight loss goals.

One thing that you can do if you are interested and want more accurate numbers to work with is to go visit your doctor. Your doctor will be able to perform blood work on you in order to see if you are short on any vital minerals or nutrients and they will also be able to do tests in order to get a fairly accurate number as to the percent of body fat that you have.

Once you finally know how many calories you burn on a daily basis the next important thing is going to be, to make sure that you set a reasonable goal for yourself. It is not going to be possible to have a six pack of abs in 21 days unless you are already almost there. Just be reasonable with yourself and realize that a 1-3 pound goal each and every week depending on what kind of an effort you are putting in, is quite a reasonable goal to have.

Due to the fact one pound of weight loss is the equivalent of roughly 3500 calories; cutting 500 calories a day from your diet or adding 500 calories worth of exercise onto your schedule will allow you to lose 1 pound.

So long as you are maintaining a proper balanced diet that is equal in calories to the amount you naturally burn, you will lose that one pound of weight each week.

Even a one pound a week weight loss goal can be difficult to achieve especially if your body is fairly fit to begin with. You don't want to starve your body of food and you want to make sure that your body is getting all of the nutrients that it needs. Eating healthy foods that have essentially almost no calories is a great way to fill up after or as a part of a meal.

To give you some examples as to the types of food that are low in calories and great for filling you up, here is a small list: Broccoli, celery, carrots, cauliflower, kale, spinach, romaine lettuce, peppers, turnip, apples, pears, oranges and bananas.

Pretty much any fruits or vegetables that you can find at your local super market will help to fill you up and they won't contain a ton of calories or at least not as many as you would find in processed food.

Generally speaking, eating fruits and veggies is the best for you when they are raw. Often times boiling your vegetables or frying them up, will decrease the amount of nutrition that they have to offer which is something that you should keep in mind.

Getting into the finer details of things, nutrition is key to your health and well-being. There are two types of minerals that your body needs in order to be able to function properly. The first type is a macro mineral and the second are trace minerals.

One of the best ways to hack healthy eating is to make sure that you know which of the ingredients on a nutrition label are the most important for your body.

To help you with this task we have created a list of the common macro minerals and micro minerals that you will find in food and what they do to your body.

Macro Minerals

- **Chloride:** This macro mineral is essential to keep your fluid levels in your body in balance. The mineral helps with a lot of important factors in your body such as maintaining your blood pressure, the amount of blood and the pH in your body as well. This mineral is found in table salt and foods like lettuce and tomatoes.

- **Potassium:** This mineral is an essential tool for your muscles to contract properly. Potassium helps to maintain mineral balances in your body and even assists your body in maintaining things like blood pressure by negating the effects of sodium in your body. Potassium is found in all kinds of different fruits including: bananas, bok choy and beets.

- **Calcium:** This mineral is essential for building bones, but what a lot of people don't know about calcium is that it also helps our blood be able to clot which is essential for healing injuries. Calcium is a prominent mineral in

- **Sodium:** The main thing you need to know about sodium is that it gets absorbed into the blood. Sodium helps to regulate blood pressure. It is important to be aware that if you eat too much sodium, your body could potentially hold onto more water than normal.

- **Sulfur:** This mineral is essential for creating proteins and amino acids for the various cells and tissues that are in your body. You will find sulfur in things like oil, dairy and turnips.

- **Magnesium:** this mineral is essential to have in your body in order to produce energy. Additionally, magnesium is important for a variety of bodily functions including things like protein synthesis and controlling the glucose levels of your blood properly. You can find magnesium in things like: nuts, yogurt and things like bananas and avocadoes.

- **Phosphorus:** This mineral is commonly found in bones of your body. Like calcium, it is essential for your bones. Additionally, this mineral helps to regulate calcium in your body. You will find phosphorus in foods like meat, nuts and beans.

Micro Minerals

- **Iron:** Especially when you are doing a lot of exercise, iron is a very important mineral to have. You will find iron in food like meat, chick peas and even some cereals on the market.

- **Iodine:** Your body needs iodine in order to produce thyroid hormones. Thyroid hormones are essential for a proper, balanced metabolism. You will find iodine in foods such as: dairy products, sea food and most plants.

- **Zinc:** This is a very important mineral in your body that helps to keep your immune system in check and even assists in making sure that you have a sense of smell. You will find zinc in things like different kinds of nuts, cereals and beans.

- **Selenium:** Similar to iodine, if you want to help out your thyroid you will want to consumer selenium. Selenium has the added bonus of helping out your immune system and you can find it in a lot of foods, especially in veggies that are green in color and nuts.

- **Manganese:** This mineral is essential for your body to form itself together. It is present in forming tissues, bones, blood clots and even plays a role in sexual hormones in the body. To get manganese into your diet some of the things you should eat include: fruits, anything that is whole grain and even things like nuts.

- **Chromium:** If you are having a difficult time with digestion then chromium could be of assistance. You will find chromium in things like: potatoes, spices and fruits and veggies.

- **Fluoride:** If you have this mineral in the right quantities it can help the body to be able to maintain bone structure. You will find fluoride in all kinds of food these days, but it is definitely something to watch your intake levels on as they can cause things like dental fluorosis. Food you will find fluoride in are: fruits, veggies and a lot of kinds of dairy products.

- **Molybdenum:** This precious mineral helps to break down enzymes in the body and even helps to break down amino acids in the body. You will find molybdenum in: dairy products, nuts and a variety of meats and vegetables.

If you are having a hard time eating all of the nutrients that your body needs, always keep in mind that there are lots of nutrition supplements available on the market. There are all sorts of things that you can take ranging from things like iron supplements, potassium vitamin C etc.

Some supplements that are available will likely have some conditions on them and it is always important to read the label before purchasing. It is never a bad idea to consult with your doctor as well before you try out some new kind of medication or supplement.

It is not only unsafe for your body to lose weight at an extremely rapid pace, but it also makes it much easier to gain back. When cutting calories that hard and then switching back to eating normally again, your body will try to store as much of the excess calories that it can as fat because it will naturally worry about a possible "starvation period" happening again.

Once you have your goal set the next step is crucial. You are going to have to keep track of not only what you eat on a daily basis, but also how much you eat and how many calories that is.

Without accurately keeping track of your daily intake it is going to be next to impossible to accurately assume that you have lost weight for that day; each and every day you should be losing body fat if you stick to your calorie goals so long as you took accurate measurements of your daily activity and the natural amount of calories that your body type burns.

It is important to realize that if you are doing a hard calorie cut and you are trying to lose a lot of weight at one time, another thing your body is going to use to fuel itself is muscle.

Your body will turn to the easiest source that it has in order to fuel itself and especially if you are cutting hard just be aware that you may lose some muscle during this process.

It is important to realize that muscle is always easier to get the second time around so you shouldn't be too worried about this as it is just part of the process.

Your muscles will show through much better once you remove excess body fat anyways, which is something to keep in your mind.

Chapter 2

Losing the Weight - Week 1

During this first week, you will start to notice a lot of changes in your lifestyle. It is important that you start right from the get go, so that you can get in a routine and continue to lose weight right from the first day of the program.

The most important thing you are going to have to do is find yourself a way that you can keep track of the calories that you are eating. Some people like to do this with a notepad and others like to download fitness apps in order to keep track of their calories.

If you are just getting started with your healthy eating then there are lots of things that you can do in order to improve your kitchen cupboards to help encourage you to lose weight faster.

One of the easiest things that you can do is to throw out all of the junk in your cupboard and replace it with healthier alternatives. This includes things like cereal which can be replaced with fruit, yogurt, whole wheat bread and healthy things like oats, wheat and nuts.

Getting rid of unhealthy food in your household can really help to reduce the amount of sugar cravings that you have. Canned soups and mixes are another thing that you should consider replacing as it will be much healthier to make your own soup and create your own soup broth.

You would be surprised as to how many preservatives are used in canned goods as well as how much sodium; which isn't good for your body in bulk, is used when canning goods.

Learning to be able to track calories for homemade foods can be a challenge at first. It is really as simple as breaking down the ingredients that are in the food you are eating and then determining the portion size that you are eating in order to come up with how many calories you are consuming.

Although marking down the calories of a single ingredient in a recipe may seem like a task that is a little picky and maybe even over the top, it really isn't.

Especially in a large recipe there could be countless ingredients which can lead to a really high amount of calories in the recipe, even though it may only seem like you are putting in a small amount.

There are certainly benefits to using online fitness apps as many of these apps actually allow you to add home cooked meals and recipes into the app and therefore into your tracking software so that you can simply click on the recipe when you make the recipe again on a later date and track your calories much easier.

I suggest that you keep all of your tracking in one place, no matter whether it is in a fitness app or some kind of a fitness book that you write in. Keeping them all in one place will allow you to stay organized and keep all of your homemade recipes as well as the amount of calories within them all in one place.

Soon enough you will know exactly how many calories are in all of your main homemade dishes and it will allow you to record your portion size and the amount of calories that you ate at a much faster speed. Beyond making sure that you are tracking your calories properly, the next thing that you are going to do is make sure that you cook yourself a nice healthy breakfast each and every morning. Make sure that during this time you also prepare some healthy snacks that you can eat throughout the rest of your day.

To help you come up with some ways that you can eat better, we have created a list of eating hacks that you can use in order to help you eat less calories and lose weight at a faster pace. Here is the list:

- Instead of drenching your salad in a fatty caesar or ranch dressing, try out natural oils instead as they will be much lower in calories

- Instead of eating sugary cereals for breakfast, try eating fruits or whole grain bread products to keep you fill and get your body more vitamins and minerals

- Rather than drinking sugary drinks, try drinking water or tea instead

- If you are baking with white sugar, try replacing it with a more natural and mineral rich type of sugar such as coconut sugar

- Rather than smothering your toast or bread product in something fatty or sugary, try something more natural such as: fruit jam, hummus, or low fat cottage cheese

- Avoid foods that have anything close to 40% or above, of your daily fat intake. These foods are likely extremely unhealthy and they may not even be that filling

- Try eating your foods without smothering them in sauce. You would be surprised how much sugar and calories are loaded into things like BBQ sauce and ketchup

- Try switching your fatty frozen desserts out of your fridge and switch them for things like frozen fruit, or frozen yogurt; these are a much healthier option

- Instead of opting for a big dessert, try and eat a 2nd course of the main meal as it likely has a lot less calories in it and it also is likely to contain a lot more of the minerals and vitamins that your body needs to thrive

- If you are looking for a movie snack, try popcorn out rather than chips. Not only will you save in calories, but you would be surprised as to how much popcorn you can eat for minimal calories so long as you pop it yourself and don't smother it in butter

- If you have unhealthy food in your household left before you started this challenge, it is likely that you like this food too much to get rid of it; try and find alternatives in the marketplace and you might be surprised by what you find

When you start off eating a large breakfast, it keeps you nice and full for a much longer period of time than if you just had a small breakfast or a few snacks in the morning. Breakfast has the added bonus of allowing our body's more time to be able to process all of the calories that we eat instead of storing them as body fat.

Having access to healthy snacks throughout the duration of your day is key to keeping your weight off. When someone offers you an unhealthy snack, which is likely to happen, you can turn to your healthy snack alternative and eat this instead.

Not only will healthy snacks throughout your day cause you to eat less food during meal time, it will also keep your daily calories down and help to provide the nutrients that you need to survive and thrive.

One thing that you might not have thought much about in the past is how bad some drinks are for you. There are actually a lot of soft drinks available on the market that contain more than the daily recommended sugar intake within the serving.

It is always important to realize that sugary drinks are pretty much pointless calories as you can just drink water in order to hydrate yourself properly.

It is important to look up a huge variety of healthy snack recipes if you don't think that healthy food tastes good. There are all kinds of delicious things that you can make and some of them taste just as good if not better than the unhealthy alternative.

Always remember that you can eat unhealthy food at times, this is not part of your life that has to be unfulfilled.

Just make sure that you eat a reasonable portion of it and make sure that the rest of the food that you eat during that day corresponds to the amount of calories that you ate.

I hope that you are enjoying this book so far, and if you could spare 30 seconds, I would greatly appreciate you leaving a review on Amazon.com.

Chapter 3

The Procedure

At the end of each and every day throughout your week you will need to tally up your calories in order to see if you met your calories goal.

Many people like to make a running tally throughout their day or they like to set themselves a calorie limit for each of the meals and snacks that they eat throughout their day so that they can be sure that they met their goal at the end of the day.

A lot of people like to plan their meals and snacks for each day of the week. The nice thing about planning your meals is that you can stay under your calorie goal and you don't have to think about what you can eat, you simply just eat it.

The bad thing about this method is that you likely don't know what all you are going to be doing each and every day of the week so it can be hard to plan for surprise treats and food that you might run into throughout your daily travels. Always remember that even if you are having a hard time staying under your daily allowed calories, you can actually burn off the extra calories through physical activity.

Just because you burn off 2500 calories a day and tend to eat 3000 calories a day doesn't mean you can't lose weight. You simply need to perform 500 calories worth of exercise or do a combination of a bit of cutting combined with exercise in order to lose weight.

It is extremely important to make sure that you keep track of each and every ingredient in the meals that you make so that you can keep an accurate tally. Failing to have just one ingredient especially if it is high in sugar or fat could result in you missing your daily calorie goal without you realizing it.

Having one off day isn't the end of the world, but just realize that you are going to have to work harder every other day of the week in order to make up for that one off day.

It is always good to think about whether the temporary enjoyment we get from eating more than our daily calorie's worth of food, is really worth the excess fat we are putting onto and into our bodies.

Once you have hit the end of each and every day, or at some point during the day you need to step onto the scale in order to see what kind of progress you have made. Be aware that the amount of fluid and food in our bodies can really make your weight fluctuate quite a bit and it can be hard to tell if your weight loss is accurate.

If you want the most accurate results possible it is a good idea to weigh yourself at the same time each and every day preferably in the morning or at night so that you have roughly the same amount of water and food in your system. Get in the habit of recording your weight loss or weight gain for each day.

One of, if not the most important things to do when it comes to weight loss is to make sure that you monitor your progress and make changes accordingly.

If by your records, you believe that you should have lost 3 pounds during the week and you only lost one pound or something like a half a pound; your body likely isn't burning as many calories naturally as you originally thought and it may be a good idea to change up your macros or to lower your daily caloric intake accordingly to adjust for the new data.

Another thing that you can do if you are noticing that you aren't losing the amount of weight that you thought you were going to lose, is to exercise the amount of extra calories that you need to each and every day throughout your week.

Dividing up your exercise throughout your week is great for your heart as well as your lungs and it has the added bonus of helping you burn calories for each and every day that you exercise. Your heart actually keeps beating at a faster pace after exercising hard for even a short period of time. It is highly likely that if you were exercising pretty intensely for a while, you burned calories no only just during the exercise, but also in the hours following the exercise when your heart was beating at a faster rate.

There are roughly 3500 calories in every pound and to put that into perspective for you that will take an average person who weighs just over 150 pounds around six hours of jogging in order to burn that many calories.

The same person would have to walk for a total of 20 hours in order to lose one pound. This may seem like a lot of work just to lose one pound, but dividing that up between calories and jogging it doesn't seem so bad.

Here is an example of how you could potentially lose one pound: you could cut 500 calories each day of the week from what you eat to maintain your weight. Another thing that you could do is cut say 250 calories by eating less and cut an additional 250 calories by jogging for roughly 26 minutes a day (150-pound person) which seems like a much more reasonable amount.

There are all kinds of different activities that you can do in order to burn calories and by no means does it have to seem like you are working in order to burn calories. There are plenty of sports and games that you can play that require a high degree of skill and that can be a lot of fun to play, all while burning a ton of calories. To give you a few examples thins like: hockey, volleyball, swimming, lacrosse, baseball, taking your dog for a walk, biking and golf.

There is no perfect exercise solution for everyone, but if you are unsure as to what sorts of things you might like to do, it is a good idea to pick up your local paper, listen to your local radio station etc. and see what kinds of things are going on in the area that you live. You may be surprised as to the amount of people that you meet as well as the numerous events that go on in your local area that you weren't aware of before.

If you choose to go more aggressive and begin to work out, it is important to realize that doing so is going to cause you to burn a lot more calories as more muscle does increase your metabolism over time. If you want to get more muscle it is recommended to take in more protein as this will help you with muscle recovery as well as muscle building.

Due to one pound being a fairly high amount of calories, it is always a good idea to incorporate exercise into your daily routine. When exercise is combined with cutting calories it makes weight loss that much easier. Just remember that high intensity training will most definitely burn more calories and you can check online for the most part as to what types of activities burn how many calories or at least get a general idea that you can use.

Chapter 4

Reviewing Week One

At the end of your first week of attempting to lose weight hopefully you have started to see results on the scale. If you haven't seen any kind of a result on the scale you may need to perform additional cutting, you may be weighing yourself at a bad time or you may not have accounted for your calories properly somehow throughout the duration of your week.

At the end of this week it is important to make sure that you are starting to develop some kind of a habit that allows you to record your meals properly.

If you find that a pencil and a pad of paper aren't working to well for you, you could try keeping the info on a note on your phone or on one of the many fitness apps that are available in the marketplace.

This first week probably wasn't easy for you as cutting calories by means of taking sugary drinks and keeping an eye on the junk food and the portions of junk food that you eat is not easy.

You will likely be tempted to stuff your face with junk food on a daily basis especially if that is what everyone around you is doing. Always remember that the earlier in the day you eat a bunch of calories, the longer your body has to try and burn those calories off before you go to sleep.

Before you move onto this second week, take a look at all of the food that you ate. There are likely some things on this list that you now regret eating as they are likely unhealthy, pointless calories and probably contain a lot of sugar or fat. Moving into this next week your goal is not to eat those exact foods that you are looking at and instead supplement them with a healthier version of the same food.

No matter the food that you ate, there are tons of recipes available online and you will be surprised when you find yourself a low-calorie dessert that tastes even better than the original, but I guarantee you that this will happen if you keep looking and continue to try out new things.

Eventually you may even try to come up with your own recipes and this is when you know you are well on your way to a healthier lifestyle.

Once again, thank you for reading this book, and I hope you're getting a lot of valuable information. I would greatly appreciate it if you could take 30 seconds to leave me a review for this book on Amazon.com.

Enjoying this book?

Check out our other best sellers!

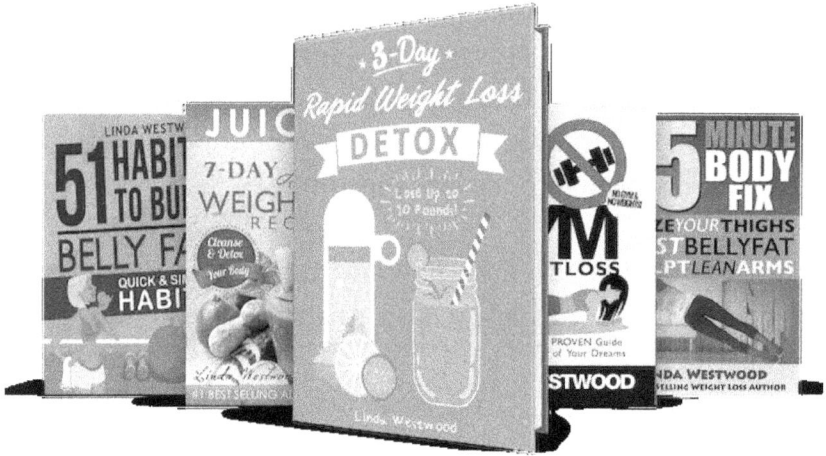

Get your next book on sale here:

TopFitnessAdvice.com/go/books

Chapter 5

Losing the Weight - Week 2

During this week, you should notice that you begin to set yourself into some kind of a routine. You should be getting up at a decent time, preparing snacks for yourself and counting each and every calorie that you eat.

The next step that you need to take in order to lose your weight as fast as you can is to change the actual food that you are eating.

There is a reason why the first week had you eating all of your regular foods, this allowed you to get comfortable with the program, and get counting calories for the food that you were eating.

There are things other than just minerals that you should pay attention to on the back of product packaging. One of the most important things to take a look at are the daily vitamins that your body needs. These include:

- **Vitamin A:** This fat-soluble vitamin is needed in your body in order to grow and for developing cells. The vitamin can be found in things like: fish and dairy products.

- **Vitamin D:** This fat-soluble vitamin is needed in your body to allow it to be able to absorb calcium. Without vitamin D, you would be able to have strong bones and teeth. You can find vitamin D in foods like: fish, dairy products and your body actually makes vitamin D when you are in the sun.

- **Vitamin E:** This fat-soluble vitamin is needed in your body in order for it to be able to maintain your red blood cell count. Additionally, vitamin E helps your body be able to maintain your muscle structure. You can find vitamin E in foods like: vegetables, nuts and dairy products.

- **Vitamin K:** This fat-soluble vitamin is needed in your body in order for it to be able to clot blood properly. Vitamin K is most commonly found in green veggies and you will be able to get a lot of it by eating things like: broccoli, spinach and even something like liver.

- **Vitamin C:** This water-soluble vitamin is needed in order for your body to be able to heal injuries, absorb iron and improve the strength of blood vessels. You can find vitamin C in a lot of citrus fruit, but you will also find it in veggies and many kinds of juice.

- **Thiamine B1:** This water-soluble vitamin is needed in order to maintain your metabolism and to keep up your energy levels. Additionally, B1 helps you be able to digest food and even helps the nerves in your body be able to function correctly. You can find this type of vitamin in: nuts, meat and many kinds of cereals.

- **Riboflavin B2:** This water-soluble vitamin helps your body be able to maintain healthy skin and good eyes. To add to that, this vitamin also helps your energy levels as well as your metabolism. This vitamin can be found in things like rice, cereal and dairy products.

- **Niacin B3:** This water-soluble vitamin helps the body be able to grow properly. The vitamin is known to be able to lower cholesterol levels and is needed to help metabolize energy as well. You can find B3 in foods like: dairy, meats and beans.

- **Pantothenic Acid B5:** This water-soluble vitamin helps your energy levels, your metabolism and helps to make your blood sugar levels normal. The best thing about B5 is that it is in almost all foods that you eat.

- **Pyroxidine B6:** This water-soluble vitamin helps your body be able to break protein down. Additionally, B6 helps your nerves be able to function properly and helps with synthesis of red blood cells.

- **Biotin B7:** This water-soluble vitamin is essential in order for your body to have proper energy levels and to have a healthy, normal metabolism. You can find B7 in things like beans, dairy and nuts.

- **Folate B9:** This water-soluble vitamin is needed for your body to be able to make DNA the right way. B9 makes red blood cells and helps to synthesize amino acids. You will find vitamin B9 in things like: flour, avocados, and yeast.

- **Cobalamin B12:** This water-soluble vitamin is used in your body in order to help create red blood cells and

DNA. In order to get B12 in your diet all you have to do is consume animal products as they all have B12.

Besides vitamins, one thing that you probably noticed when you were eating, is that below the calories on the package, there were a variety of other nutrition facts on the package that had percent of daily value next to them.

This is our next focus and topic and the next most important thing that you are going to want to pay attention to when you are choosing foods to eat. The most important thing to realize about nutrition labels is that the portion size will be on the label and you should always read this before assuming that it refers to the full contents of the package.

The thing about a nutrition label is that they are all based around the average 2000 calorie diet, so unless you burn 2000 calories exactly on a daily basis then the nutrition percentages are not dead on for you. They will, however, give you a good grasp as to how healthy the product actually is.

Generally speaking, food is broken down into three different categories. These categories include: carbs, protein and fat.

Each and every day you will not only want to try and meet your calorie goals, but you will also want to try and meet your daily values for the percent of calories that you get from each of these three categories.

Carbs are the portion of your diet that you should be getting the most amount of. It is recommended that a person get between 45-65 percent of their daily calories as a result of eating carbs.

Generally speaking, reducing the amount of carbs in your diet is one of the best ways that you can lose weight.

Low carb diets are great as they allow you to have low blood sugar and it actually reduces your appetite which allows you to be able to eat less and stay full. Going on a low carb diet reduces the amount of sugar and starches that you intake, which can be hard to break down and often get stored as fat, and replaces these with fat or protein accordingly.

Another diet that many people like to try is a diet that is low in fat. It is generally recommended that you intake between 20 to 35 percent of your daily caloric intake with fat.

Your body needs fat in order to survive so you can't cut fat entirely out of your diet. Fat unfortunately has the most calories of all nutrients so you will really have to watch what you eat in order to stay under the daily percentages.

You should have between 10 to 35 percent of your total calories from eating protein. As you can see there is a really broad spectrum recommended for each of these three nutrients because there are so many theories as to which diet is the healthiest for our bodies and no one truly knows the answer.

Fortunately, a lot of research has been done and generally speaking in order to get the maximum amount of weight loss, protein carries the most metabolic benefits of the three nutrients.

So if you are trying to pick your daily percentages, and hack your nutrition, it may be a good idea to cut carbs or fat and exchange them for protein whenever possible so long as you are staying in the daily recommended percentage ranges.

Remember that it is always a good idea to have a discussion with your doctor about your diet as there is no perfect diet for everyone.

Especially if you have something like diabetes it can be hard to change up your diet without greatly affecting your blood sugar levels and you may have to go for a long-term change rather than short term so that your body has a chance to adapt.

Another thing that you may want to consider this week is adjusting your goals.

Depending on how hard you went the first week, you could be down a substantial amount of weight. However, if you are feeling like you lost too much weight or you feel as though you didn't lose enough weight it is important to change up your daily caloric intake and change your goals accordingly.

By no means are you in a race in order to see if you can lose weight the fastest. It is not easy to lose weight and you will have to put a lot of time and effort in so that you can have your "ideal" body. You will also have to put a lot of work in just to keep the body that you want, once you get to that stage in time.

The entire weight loss process can take a long time and it is your lifestyle that will affect how long this process takes as well as your starting weight.

For some people a combination of eating healthy and doing lots of activities can take some getting used to and can be a huge lifestyle change that gradually happens over time.

It is important not to push yourself so hard that you wear yourself out, but it is important to push yourself hard enough that you continue to progress towards your goals.

Chapter 6

Reviewing Week Two

At the end of this week it is important to make sure that you really look into your progress in order to make sure that you are still on track. If you are skipping recording meals and snacks you are only cheating yourself.

Monitoring your calories is the only sure way to make sure that you are maintaining, losing or gaining weight and therefore no matter whether you are done losing the weight that you want to lose, or if you still have a ton of weight left to lose then you should still be doing this on a daily basis.

Heading into week three, you are already well on your way to a healthier lifestyle if you have been following this guide. It is important to step back and have another look at your progress in order to see how things are progressing.

If it turns out that you lost weight during this week, add up your total calories for the week and subtract that number by seven times the amount of calories that you think you burn on a daily basis. Check to see whether the amount of calories matches the amount of weight that you lost. If you want to hack your way to weight loss, keep in mind that one pound is roughly 3500 calories.

If you find that your number was too high or a little too low then you may not be recording calories with a hundred percent accuracy. If it only a little bit off of the point then you can be pretty certain that you were doing a good job as often times you will have to estimate your portion sizes and they won't always be a hundred percent accurate.

It is also a good time to reflect back on the activities that you did throughout the week and determine which ones were your favorites. Some events do require you to book ahead so make sure that you don't miss out on one of your favorite activities as a result of not getting prepared properly for week three.

Heading into the final week of this challenge we have one final goal for you. This goal is not to go hard exercising or dieting or anything like that. This goal is for you to make some more modifications to your diet.

Try some new foods, some new snacks, eat more food in the morning and spread out your calories throughout your day; the key to hacking nutrition and to keep the weight off for good is to incorporate this into your life all while maintaining your regular routine.

Others who are considering purchasing this book would love to know what you think. If you could spare a few seconds, they would greatly appreciate reading an honest review from you. Simply visit the page on Amazon.com.

Chapter 7

Losing the Weight - Week 3

During week three the most important thing that you can do is monitor your progress. The further you get into this program/lifestyle instead of tapering off at the end, you need to make this a part of your new life. Week three is all about the little things, but it is also about remembering the big picture and sticking with your goals.

It is important to stick in your head that when you are going into week three of healthy eating, you shouldn't think of this as week three of your diet; instead you should think of this as week three of your new and improved life.

By losing excess fat, your body is less prone to getting things like diseases and cancer. You will also be less at risk to things like strokes and heart attacks. Especially if you combine a healthy exercise routine along with your healthy eating habits you are setting yourself up for a lifetime of good health.

You need to make sure that your "new diet" is meeting all of your body's nutrition needs and that you are getting a good amount of protein, fat and carbs so that you can maintain a healthy lifestyle.

Some apps that you can use will tell you the exact amount of protein, carbs and fat that are in your diet and some apps are even programmed to send you notifications in order to remind you to log the food that you are supposed to eat.

When you reach for that extra cookie just realize that you really are sacrificing a small portion of your good health during that day and thinking in this fashion can really help to get you eating healthier on a consistent basis.

The best thing about healthy foods like fruits and veggies is that they are fairly minimal in calories, to hack your nutrition you need to replace the bad foods in your diet with these instead.

When you are eating your healthy snacks, it is always best to eat them plain and without dressing whenever possible as many of them are high in fat and sugar content.

Fruit is naturally high in sugar to begin with so it is quite important for your blood sugar and health to get either light dressings or to stay away from them when possible.

During this week try to try out some new things. Try some new foods out and even try out some new physical activities. Trying new things out allows you to have the opportunity to find new favorite foods which you can use to replace and destroy your old eating habits.

You may find new favorite sports and activities that you can do in order to help you lose excess weight at a faster pace. Going out and trying new things also allows you to meet new people and can be a great social experience.

It is important to keep in mind that not matter your results over the last three weeks, all isn't the end of the world if you didn't lose much or any weight during this process. This simply means that you need to cut harder or that you should throw a little bit more exercise into your routine in order to help you lose the weight that you desire.

Losing weight is by no means something that is easy to do and it is by no means an easy task to change your lifestyle in as little as three weeks. Think of this 21-day challenge as a stepping stone to your good health and well-being and that there are plenty more sacrifices and fun things that you can do in your life all while maintaining a healthy, well balanced diet.

During this week, try to throw out or donate all of that extra food that you no longer want to eat in your healthy and more active lifestyle. Not only will this allow you to be able to put new, healthier alternatives in your cupboard, but it will also be a good way to try and keep you from falling back into your old unhealthy eating habits.

Chapter 8

Reviewing Week Three

At the end of this week this is where you should start to see progress being made. At this point you have been tracking calories for 21 full days for each and every meal that you eat.

Not only that, but I bet you have also started to check the nutrition label for things like sugar, fat and sodium in order to get an idea as to how unhealthy the product really is that you are eating.

This stepping stone is a good teller that you are well on your way to hacking nutrition and healthy eating as well as keeping the weight off that you lose for good.

Many of the things that you eat will likely surprise you if you have never looked at the ingredients before. There can be a lot of calories in some pretty small food items and you can eat a lot more food if you instead buy some healthier alternatives.

Since this is just the beginning of your new lifestyle, it is important to use these three weeks as a referencing point. See how much progress you made and think about how much you want to lose the excess weight that you have.

To put things into perspective for you it can take some people up to a year or even more of counting calories and cutting and exercising before they get to the weight that they want to be.

If you really want to lose weight you are definitely going to have to work hard for it and you are definitely going to have to monitor your progress on a consistent basis.

Often times even when you are cutting calories you may see that your body plateaus and stops losing weight; this is a sign that your body has possibly adjusted its metabolism to support your new body, or that you need to cut more calories or exercise harder in order to lose more weight.

Generally, after losing a lot of weight, it only becomes more difficult over time. Our bodies are built to use fat as a backup source of energy and it can be hard to force them to be able to use this energy especially when the reserves are getting low.

With continued work, you will lose the weight that you want to and you can move onto trying to maintain a balance. In order to help you, we have come up with some tips.

I hope you have learned something from this book so far and would greatly appreciate it if you could leave an honest review on Amazon.com.

Chapter 9

Maintaining A Balance

This is by far the most difficult part of the entire procedure. After you have lost the weight that you wanted to lose, many people go back to their old lifestyles and end up putting back on the weight that they lost within as little as a few months' time.

In order to keep the weight off, you will have to find the exact amount of calories that you can eat on a daily basis in order to stay at the same weight. It can take quite some time before learning this number and you definitely won't need to weigh yourself on a daily basis once you think you are close.

After about 4-5 weeks of checking your numbers on the same day each week and checking out the daily calories that you ate during each of those weeks you should be able to get a good grasp as to the amount of calories that you should eat on a daily basis.

One of the main problems you might encounter when trying to find your balance is that the amount of physical activity that you do on a daily basis may vary a lot depending on the day. It is important to figure out about how many calories you burned while performing your physical activity and supplement the extra calories into your eating throughout your day.

Another thing that can throw off your healthy weight is sickness. It is important to realize that at any point in time you could come down with an illness that could prevent you from being your energetic self. Most of the time when a person is sick they lose some of their appetite and often don't feel like working out as this makes them even sicker.

One of the best things you can do to start to become better when you come down with a cold is to eat healthy and make sure that you get a lot of sleep.

Remember that even though you may come out of a cold weighing less than you did before, it is not hard to put weight back on to get back to a healthy body; just make sure that you put it on gradually and healthily and don't pound back three bags of chips just to try and get your weight back up to par.

You may lose some muscle mass during sickness and periods of dieting and this is likely something that you don't really want to lose.

In order to be able to maintain your muscles and lose weight at the same time it is a good idea to perform a variety of bodily exercises on a daily basis.

If you find that you are unable to perform much in the way of body exercises, just do what you can as some exercise is always better than no exercise at all.

It is important to find your own balance between eating healthy and unhealthy foods as no method is perfect for everyone.

There is no one on the planet for the most part who doesn't enjoy a nice treat every once and a while and it is important to find a way to incorporate these things into your diet so that you are still getting all of the nutrition that your body needs and so that you can make sure that you aren't going overboard on things like fat and sugar.

There are several ways that you can slip a treat into your diet. One great way of eating treats is managing your portion size; this hack will allow you to have a treat, a small one, on a daily basis if you like.

Another way you can sneak a treat into your diet is by cutting a few calories out of each of your meals in order to account for the snack that is higher in calories. Dividing up the calories into three meals will allow you to still have a decent size meal and you won't have to feel as guilty about eating that special treat.

Another thing that you can do which helps some people out is to set some kind of a limit on the amount of unhealthy snacks during the period of a week.

This can give you peace of mind knowing that these are available to you throughout your week whenever you feel like it; it is just important to make sure that you adapt your diet accordingly so that you meet your calories goals.

It is often said that money can be an issue when it comes to eating healthily. Healthy food is said to cost more than that of junk food and this means that you may have to stretch your budget a little further when you are buying groceries.

It is a good idea to hack healthy eating and look at portion sizes when you are shopping. Some fruits and vegetables are much larger than other ones for the same relative price.

Fruits and vegetables do go bad over time unlike junk food so it can be smart to only buy for 3-5 days at a time. This will allow you to better plan your meals and give you a bit of flexibility as to what you will be eating later on in the week. Always make sure that your fridge is set on the right settings or you may find that your produce rots faster than it should.

Chapter 10

Lifestyle Change

If you want to live a long and happy life, not only are you going to have to consider this plan for yourself as a lifestyle, but you are going to have to stick to it.

Maintaining healthy eating choices and matching your daily caloric intake with that of your body is essential for you in order to be able to maintain your body weight.

If you are not willing to change your lifestyle not only are you going to gain any of the weight that you lost back on, but you are also going to be more at risk for nutrition deficiencies and diseases like diabetes.

Keeping poor food out of your household and filling it with healthy alternatives is one of the best ways that you can keep yourself on track.

There are so many foods that you can try out and there are so many recipes that are great alternatives to unhealthy foods. It is a good idea to find yourself a nice recipe app especially if before this guide you haven't done a ton of healthy eating in the past.

Always remember that it is a good idea to have a consultation with your doctor every once and a while especially when you are feeling ill. You would be surprised as to just how many headaches and illnesses are caused by improper nutrition and that they can easily be fixed by eating in a proper manner.

Always remember that even if you don't know the exact amount of calories that you need or what you relatively burn on a daily basis, you can always look things up online and get a very good general idea. Online resources are a great way to learn new recipes and to get motivation to keep working hard in order to meet your weight loss goals.

Keep in mind that although you are trying to maintain a healthy lifestyle, this does not mean that you have to skip out on meals with friends and family at restaurants etc.

There are all kinds of healthy options at these places that you likely aren't aware of and you can always ask the waitress or have a look at the menu in order to find out the amount of calories that are in each of the dishes so that you can make a more informed decision for yourself.

Make sure that you take your tracking device or paper with you wherever you go unless you are one of those people with a really good memory who does it at the end of each day.

It can be very difficult to remember the amount of calories that were in each of the items that you ate throughout your day and having your device or note pad on you at all times will make it a lot less stressful for you and allow you to write down your calories whenever you need.

Often times when people start to track their calories and they get into some kind of a routine with it, they begin to realize that other parts of their diet are lacking and will begin to supplement their diet with the proper nutrition that their body needs.

Many of the fitness apps available keep track of and have the nutrition labels of the products that you purchase already incorporated into the app. This will allow you to record the items that you have eaten at a fast rate and it will allow you to track your nutrition as well as your calories at the same time.

It is important to realize that even if you have suffered from a poor diet and an overweight body for the entire duration of your life, it can really help to increase your overall life expectancy and health and well-being by losing that excess weight that you have had for so long.

If you are extremely overweight and you end up losing a ton of weight and end up with wrinkles of fat on your stomach you can actually get surgery in order to repair these and get rid of them completely. Not only will removing the excess fat make it easier for you to get around, it will also increase blood flow to various places in your body resulting in a lower chance of things like organ failure, immobility etc.

It is consistently important that you keep some kind of a goal in mind throughout your life so that you always have something that you can work towards.

Even if you have a perfect body, your goal can be to maintain that body. There is always something out there that you can do and it is not going to be easy, but it will allow you to have a healthier life and hopefully allow you to live a longer one as well.

If you find that writing down each and every one of your calories is a pain after each meal that you eat, you can always wait until the end of the day to tally up your calories in order to see if you hit your goals. Although this definitely isn't the most efficient method as it does require you to do some guess work and adjusting, it definitely is a method that some people like to use.

If you find yourself hopping in and out of diets on a regular basis and eating all kinds of weird food, stop. Just remember that it really isn't all that important as to the actual foods that you eat.

Make sure that your body has the proper nutrients that it needs and make sure you know how many calories your body burns on a daily basis. Match or get under that amount of calories in order to lose or maintain your weight accordingly. This is how you hack healthy eating and nutrition in order to lose weight and keep it off for good.

If you find yourself fading off and you start to slide back into your old eating habits, stop. Get rid of these foods and replace them with healthier alternatives that taste almost the same. These foods are obviously something that you truly enjoy, but the thing is there is almost no junk food out there that doesn't have a similar tasting healthy alternative, all you have to do is look for one.

One thing that you may not have thought about when considering this lifestyle change is the potential for injury and how this may affect your new life. If you become injured it can really slow down your exercising and therefore it is always a good idea to be prepared to change up your calorie intake on a regular basis.

There are plenty of things that can change in one's lifestyle and it is always important to stay on top of these changes and adapt your diet accordingly. Someone who now eats 500 more calories a day can be just as healthy and just as fit as they were one year ago when they ate 500 calories less.

It is important to realize that these types of changes do occur depending on what is going on in our lives and it is likely that you won't be able to have a massive amount of exercise each and every day.

Just make sure that every week, or every couple weeks in your life you think about the amount of exercise that you have done lately and tally up the amount of calories that you have burned compared to that of weeks in the past.

Use this number in order to be able to set new more accurate calorie goals for yourself. It is quite common to see people have increased calories when they are attempting to lose weight, largely because they increase their physical activity by a lot and need more calories in order to be able to provide their body with the energy and the nutrition that they need in order to thrive.

It is often said that the people you are around the most often, are the people that have the largest influences on your lifestyle and how you are going to turn out.

It is important to realize that these influences do exist, but to take your own path to health and well-being and don't let other people influence the decisions that you make in this regard as they likely just aren't willing to put in the same amount of effort that you are in order to change their body for the better.

You don't have to eat healthy smoothies every day in order to have proper nutrition. All you have to do is input the foods you eat into some kind of a fitness app and it will tell you right away if you are deficient in something. If you don't have a fitness app or a way of using one, simply take your list of everything that you ate during the three weeks or even one week of this guide and take it to your doctor and see what they think as to whether you are lacking in any of the nutrition that your body needs in order to be healthy.

Don't forget to share your thoughts on this book by leaving a review on Amazon.com. It takes just a few seconds.

Did You Know You Are MOST Likely Burning Fat Too SLOW?

Discover The Most POWERFUL Method to Start Burning Fat Up to 400% Faster!

For this month only, you can get Bruce's best-selling & most popular book absolutely free – *The Most Powerful Method to Burn Fat Up to 400% Faster!*

Get Your FREE Copy Here:

TopFitnessAdvice.com/Download

Discover exactly what you need to do to **put your metabolism into hyperdrive** and have your **fat melt away effortlessly**. And learn the biological "hacks" that have been scientifically proven to **boost the rate that your body burns fat by up to 400%.** With this book, readers were able to reach their fitness goals significantly quicker, so it's highly recommended that you get this book, especially while it's free!

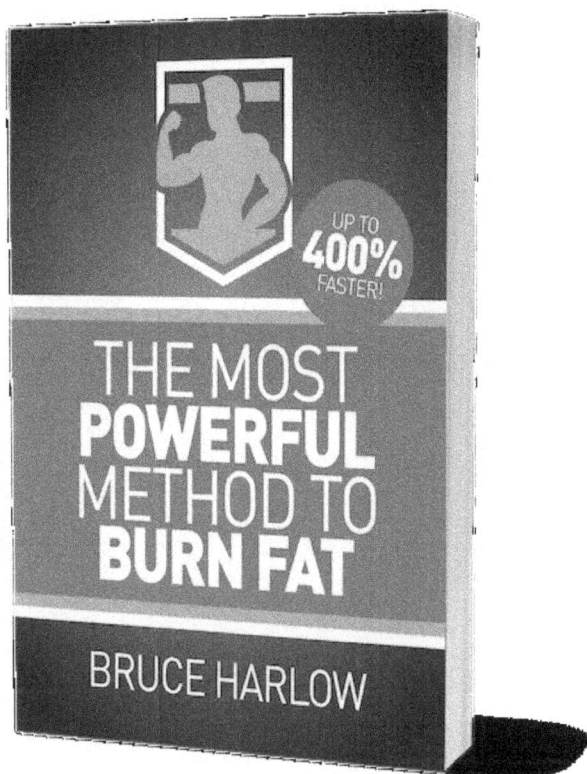

Get Your FREE Copy Here:

TopFitnessAdvice.com/Download

Conclusion

Hopefully after reading through all of the tips contained in this book you now feel like you have a better grasp on how you can hack your lifestyle to lose weight and how you can keep it off for good. It is going to take a lot of work to be able to lose the weight and it is going to take even more work in order to keep that extra weight from coming back on.

It is extremely important to make sure that you count your calories as if this is the only thing that you do in an attempt to lose weight, you will begin to lose weight once you begin to realize how many calories you tend to burn on a daily basis.

It is also extremely important to make sure that you set realistic expectations for yourself as it is generally not recommended to cut more than 1-3 pounds of body fat in a week. If you want to cut more than this you will likely be depriving your body of the nutrition that it needs or you are working your body too hard which could result in something such as a heart attack or a stroke occurring.

Whenever you are exercising it is never a bad idea to wear some kind of a heart rate monitor so that you can be sure that you are training in an appropriate heart rate area. There are all sorts of options available and it can really give you some peace of mind when you know that you are exercising at a safe rate for your body.

It is important to take both dieting as well as exercise at your own pace. Obviously if you haven't ran on a treadmill or been running before you can't be expected to suddenly run a marathon. It will take time for your body to develop and be in better physical shape, the same as it will take your body some time to develop and take advantage of your better eating habits.

You definitely may not see results right away, but it is important to keep trying. The more effort that you put in, the more likely you are to see results.

Just be reasonable, set reasonable goals for both your overall caloric intake as well as your weight loss goals and you will be well on your way towards becoming a new, healthier you.

No matter how well this program works for you it is important to realize that losing weight can take time. 3500 calories is a lot of calories to burn and it could take you as long as two to three weeks depending on your activity level if you aren't willing to do much in the way of cutting.

It is important to make sure that you have an accurate scale so that you can keep track of your weight loss accordingly, always make sure that you write down your weight so that you can reference it later and so you can track and see your progress in motion to keep you motivated.

Remember that you don't have to eat foods that you don't enjoy in order to be healthy, you simply have to eat reasonable portion sizes of the things that aren't as healthy for you and you should also consider substituting ingredients or the whole recipe in order to try a healthier alternative.

Always try to weigh yourself at the same time whenever possible so that your weight will be more accurate. Weighing yourself at different times of the day will allow water weight and food and other drink to affect how much you weigh.

You would actually be surprised as to how much clothes can weigh and even a light set of clothes can weigh as much as 2 pounds so this is important to consider whenever you are weighing in. If you want to be the most accurate for your weigh in's you may want to do it without any clothes on or just wearing some underwear.

It is important to remember that losing weight is not a contest and losing weight at too fast of a pace can actually cause harm to your body. A 1-3 pound weight loss per week is all that is recommended and even that can be pushing it depending on your body type. Make sure that you set a goal for yourself and adjust as you need.

Best of luck on your weight loss journey and hope that this guide has helped you to realize that there is no such thing as a "diet" if you want to lose weight, you have to hack into and change your lifestyle and your mindset to keep the weight off for good.

Enjoying this book?

Check out our other best sellers!

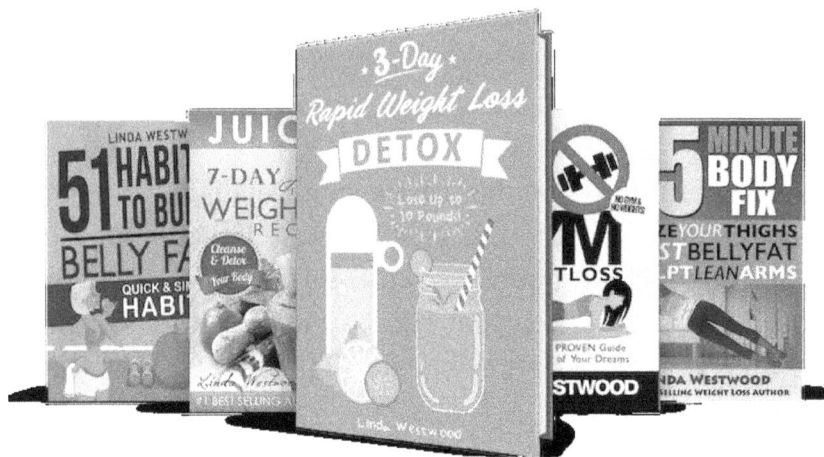

Get your next book on sale here:

TopFitnessAdvice.com/go/books

Final Words

I would like to thank you for purchasing my book and I hope I have been able to help you and educate you on something new.

If you have enjoyed this book and would like to share your positive thoughts, could you please take 30 seconds of your time to go back and give me a review on my Amazon book page.

I greatly appreciate seeing these reviews because it helps me share my hard work.

You can leave me a review on Amazon.com.

Again, thank you and I wish you all the best!

www.ingramcontent.com/pod-product-compliance
Lightning Source LLC
Chambersburg PA
CBHW031208020426
42333CB00013B/843